LOW POTASSIUM FOOD LIST FOR KIDNEY DISEASE PATIENTS

Your Essential Guide to Kidney-Friendly
Eating and Wellness

Brenda T. Fred

INTRODUCTION

Kidney disease is a serious condition that affects millions of people worldwide. For those living with kidney disease, managing potassium intake is crucial to maintaining health and preventing complications. Potassium is a mineral that plays a vital role in various bodily functions, including nerve and muscle function, but when the kidneys are not working properly, potassium can build up to dangerous levels in the blood.

This book is designed to be a comprehensive guide for kidney disease patients who need to follow a low-potassium diet. It provides a clear, organized list of foods that are low in potassium, making it easier to make safe and healthy choices. From fruits and vegetables to proteins and beverages, this guide covers a wide range of food categories to help you maintain a balanced and enjoyable diet.

Managing a low-potassium diet doesn't have to be overwhelming. With practical tips, sample meal plans, and delicious recipes, this book will empower you to take control of your health. Whether you're newly diagnosed or have been managing kidney disease for years, this guide will be an essential resource on your journey to better health.

TABLE OF CONTENTS

1.1 Understanding Kidney Disease

Kidney disease, also known as chronic kidney disease (CKD), occurs when the kidneys gradually lose their ability to function effectively over time. The kidneys are vital organs that filter waste products, excess fluids, and toxins from the blood, which are then excreted as urine. They also help regulate blood pressure, produce hormones that control red blood cell production, and balance important minerals like sodium and potassium in the body.

When the kidneys are damaged, they can no longer perform these critical functions as efficiently, leading to a buildup of waste and fluid in the body. This can result in a range of health problems, including high blood pressure, anemia, bone disease, and nerve damage. In the later stages of kidney disease, known as end-stage renal disease (ESRD), dialysis or a kidney transplant may be necessary to maintain life.

Kidney disease is often referred to as a "silent" condition because it can progress slowly without causing noticeable symptoms until the damage is significant. Early detection and management are key to slowing the progression of the disease and minimizing complications. Regular monitoring of kidney function, blood pressure, and other related health markers is essential for those at risk.

One of the critical aspects of managing kidney disease is controlling the intake of certain nutrients, particularly potassium. As the kidneys become less effective at filtering potassium, it can accumulate in the blood, leading to hyperkalemia—a condition characterized by dangerously high potassium levels. Hyperkalemia can cause symptoms like muscle weakness, fatigue, and in severe cases, life-threatening heart problems.

Understanding kidney disease and its impact on your health is the first step toward managing the condition effectively. By making informed choices about your diet, particularly with regard to potassium intake, you can play an active role in protecting your kidney function and overall well-being.

1.2 The Role of Potassium in the Body

Potassium is an essential mineral and electrolyte that plays a crucial role in maintaining the body's overall health and proper functioning. It is involved in a variety of physiological processes, making it vital for everything from muscle contractions to maintaining a stable heartbeat.

One of potassium's primary functions is to help regulate fluid balance in the body. It works closely with sodium, another key electrolyte, to control the movement of fluids in and out of cells. This balance is essential for maintaining proper cell function, blood volume, and blood pressure. Without sufficient potassium, cells may become dehydrated, or fluid imbalances may lead to high blood pressure and other cardiovascular issues.

Potassium is also critical for nerve function. It facilitates the transmission of nerve signals by generating electrical impulses that allow nerves to communicate with muscles and other tissues. This process is what enables muscles to contract and relax, making potassium essential for all types of muscle activity, including the beating of the heart. Adequate levels of potassium help ensure that your heart beats in a regular, rhythmic pattern, reducing the risk of arrhythmias and other heart-related conditions.

In addition to these functions, potassium plays a role in maintaining the body's acid-base balance, which is crucial for overall metabolic processes. It also helps support bone health by preventing the loss of calcium from bones, which can occur when potassium levels are low.

Despite its importance, potassium must be maintained within a narrow range in the blood. Both too much and too little potassium can have serious health consequences. For people with healthy kidneys, excess potassium is usually excreted in urine. However, when kidney function is impaired, the body may struggle to remove excess potassium, leading to hyperkalemia—a condition where potassium levels become dangerously high.

Hyperkalemia can cause a range of symptoms, from muscle weakness and fatigue to life-threatening cardiac events. Therefore, for individuals with kidney disease, it is particularly important to monitor and manage potassium intake to prevent complications.

Potassium is vital for many of the body's essential functions, including fluid balance, nerve transmission, muscle contractions, and heart function. Understanding the role of potassium in the body highlights why it is so important to manage potassium levels, especially for those with kidney disease. By doing so, you can help protect your overall health and reduce the risk of serious complications.

1.3 Why Managing Potassium is Crucial for Kidney Disease Patients

For individuals with kidney disease, managing potassium levels is of paramount importance due to the kidneys' reduced ability to filter and eliminate excess potassium from the body. When the kidneys are functioning normally, they regulate potassium levels by removing any surplus through urine. However, as kidney function declines, this process becomes less efficient, leading to a potential buildup of potassium in the blood, a condition known as hyperkalemia.

Hyperkalemia is particularly dangerous because it can disrupt the normal functioning of the heart and other muscles. Potassium is essential for maintaining the electrical impulses that control muscle contractions, including the heartbeat. When potassium levels become too high, it can interfere with these impulses, potentially causing severe complications such as muscle weakness, irregular heartbeats (arrhythmias), and in extreme cases, cardiac arrest.

Symptoms of hyperkalemia can range from mild, such as fatigue and muscle weakness, to severe, including chest pain, palpitations, and difficulty breathing. However, hyperkalemia can also be asymptomatic, meaning it may not produce noticeable symptoms until potassium levels are dangerously high. This makes regular monitoring and proactive management of potassium intake vital for kidney disease patients.

Diet plays a crucial role in managing potassium levels. Many common foods, especially fruits, vegetables, and some proteins, are naturally high in potassium. Without careful planning, a typical diet could easily lead to potassium intake that exceeds the safe limits for someone with impaired kidney function. By following a low-potassium diet, kidney disease patients can reduce the risk of hyperkalemia and its associated complications.

In addition to dietary management, other factors such as certain medications and medical conditions can also influence potassium levels. For instance, some blood pressure medications, which are often prescribed to kidney disease patients, can increase potassium levels. Therefore, it is essential for patients to work closely with their healthcare providers to monitor their potassium levels regularly and adjust their diet, medications, and lifestyle accordingly.

Managing potassium is not just about avoiding immediate health risks; it's also about preserving overall kidney function and quality of life. By maintaining safe potassium levels, patients can help slow the progression of kidney disease, reduce the risk of cardiovascular complications, and maintain better overall health.

Managing potassium levels is crucial for kidney disease patients because of the kidneys' diminished ability to regulate this mineral. Proper potassium management through diet, medication, and regular monitoring is essential to prevent the serious health risks associated with hyperkalemia and to support long-term kidney health.

1.4 How to Use This Low Potassium Food List

safe and healthy dietary choices. Each section categorizes foods based on their potassium content, making it easy to identify which items to include in your diet and which to limit or avoid. Use this list when planning meals, grocery shopping, or dining out to help you manage your potassium intake effectively. By incorporating these low potassium options into your daily routine, you can better control your potassium levels and support your overall health.

2. Potassium Levels in Common Foods

2.1 High Potassium Foods to Avoid

For individuals with kidney disease, avoiding high-potassium foods is essential to prevent the dangerous buildup of potassium in the blood. Many commonly consumed foods are rich in potassium, and while they may be healthy for the general population, they can pose serious risks for those with impaired kidney function.

Here are some of the primary categories of high-potassium foods to be aware of:

1. Fruits

- **Bananas:** A single banana can contain more than 400 mg of potassium, making it a fruit to avoid or limit.
- **Oranges and Orange Juice:** Both the fruit and its juice are high in potassium and should be minimized in the diet.
- **Avocados:** While avocados are nutrient-rich, they are also very high in potassium, with one avocado containing nearly 1,000 mg.
- **Cantaloupe and Honeydew Melon:** These melons are particularly high in potassium and should be limited.

2. Vegetables

- **Potatoes:** Whether baked, mashed, or fried, potatoes are high in potassium, especially if the skin is left on. Boiling can reduce potassium levels, but they should still be consumed sparingly.
- **Tomatoes and Tomato Products:** This includes fresh tomatoes, tomato sauce, and tomato juice, all of which are high in potassium.

- **Spinach and Swiss Chard:** These leafy greens, especially when cooked, are high in potassium and should be limited.
- **Squash:** Certain types of squash, particularly winter squash, are high in potassium.

3. Dairy Products

- **Milk:** Both regular and low-fat milk are high in potassium, with one cup containing over 350 mg. Alternatives like almond or rice milk (without added potassium) may be better choices.
- **Yogurt:** Many types of yogurt, particularly those with added fruits, can be high in potassium.

4. Proteins

- **Certain Fish:** Fish like salmon, tuna, and cod are high in potassium, especially in larger portions. They can still be included in the diet but should be consumed in moderation.
- **Beef and Pork:** These meats can be high in potassium, particularly in larger servings. Lean cuts may be a better option, but portion control is key.
- **Legumes:** Beans, lentils, and other legumes are protein-rich but also high in potassium. They should be limited or carefully portioned.

5. Nuts and Seeds

- **Almonds, Peanuts, and Other Nuts:** While nutritious, nuts and seeds are generally high in potassium and should be eaten in small amounts, if at all.

6. Grains and Starches

- **Bran and Whole Grains:** Whole grain breads, cereals, and bran are often high in potassium, especially when fortified. Opt for refined grains in smaller portions as they are typically lower in potassium.

7. Beverages

- **Coconut Water:** Known for its high potassium content, coconut water is a beverage to avoid.
- **Certain Sports Drinks:** Many sports drinks are fortified with potassium and should be avoided by those needing to limit their intake.

By being mindful of these high-potassium foods, you can make better dietary choices that align with your health needs. Remember, portion size also plays a significant role in managing potassium intake, so even moderate-potassium foods can become problematic if consumed in large quantities. Always consult with your healthcare provider or a dietitian for personalized advice.

2.2 Moderate Potassium Foods: Use with Caution

While high-potassium foods are best avoided for those with kidney disease, there are many foods that contain moderate levels of potassium. These foods can often be included in your diet, but they should be consumed with caution and in controlled portions to avoid exceeding your daily potassium limit. Proper portion control and balancing these foods with low-potassium options are key to managing your potassium levels effectively.

Here are some examples of moderate-potassium foods and tips for how to incorporate them into your diet safely:

1. Fruits

- **Berries (Strawberries, Blueberries, Raspberries):** These fruits are lower in potassium than bananas or oranges, but still contain moderate amounts. A half-cup serving can be a safe option when balanced with other low-potassium foods.

- **Pineapple:** Pineapple is lower in potassium compared to tropical fruits like mango or papaya, but it should still be enjoyed in moderation.
- **Apples and Pears:** These fruits contain moderate potassium levels and are best consumed in smaller portions, such as one medium apple or pear.

2. Vegetables

- **Carrots:** Raw or cooked carrots have moderate potassium content. A small serving, such as half a cup, can fit into a low-potassium diet if monitored carefully.
- **Green Beans:** Green beans are a safer vegetable choice, but they still contain moderate potassium levels, so portion control is important.
- **Cauliflower:** This versatile vegetable is moderately high in potassium, particularly when cooked. A small serving can be included in meals, especially when balanced with low-potassium ingredients.

3. Dairy Products

- **Cheese:** Certain types of cheese, such as cheddar or mozzarella, have moderate potassium levels. Limiting your portion to one ounce or less can help you enjoy these foods without overloading on potassium.
- **Cottage Cheese:** A half-cup serving of cottage cheese contains a moderate amount of potassium and can be included in your diet, but it's best to avoid larger portions.

4. Proteins

- **Chicken and Turkey:** Lean poultry, such as chicken or turkey, contains moderate potassium levels. Eating smaller portions, such as three ounces per meal, can help you keep your potassium intake within safe limits.
- **Eggs:** Eggs are another protein source with moderate potassium content. One egg or two egg whites can be a safe serving size.

- **Tofu:** Tofu provides plant-based protein and is moderately high in potassium. A small portion, such as half a cup, can be included occasionally.

5. Grains and Starches

- **White Rice:** While lower in potassium than brown rice, white rice still contains moderate levels. A serving of half a cup cooked can be a good choice when balanced with other low-potassium foods.
- **Pasta:** Pasta made from refined wheat is generally moderate in potassium. Limiting your portion to one cup cooked can help manage potassium intake.
- **Oatmeal:** Oatmeal is a nutritious option with moderate potassium levels. A half-cup serving of cooked oatmeal can be part of a kidney-friendly diet when consumed with caution.

6. Nuts and Seeds

- **Peanut Butter:** Peanut butter contains moderate potassium levels. A small portion, such as one tablespoon, can be included in your diet occasionally.
- **Pumpkin Seeds:** These seeds are moderately high in potassium. Consuming a small handful, about one tablespoon, can be safe if balanced with low-potassium foods.

7. Beverages

- **Coffee and Tea:** These beverages have moderate potassium content. Limiting intake to one cup per day can help prevent excessive potassium intake.
- **Fruit Juices (Apple, Grape):** Certain fruit juices have moderate potassium levels. Limiting your portion to half a cup can help keep potassium levels in check.

Tips for Managing Moderate-Potassium Foods:

- **Portion Control:** Be mindful of serving sizes to avoid unintentionally consuming too much potassium. Smaller portions are safer and allow for more variety in your diet.
- **Balance with Low-Potassium Foods:** Pairing moderate-potassium foods with low-potassium options helps create a balanced meal that stays within your potassium limits.
- **Monitor Your Potassium Intake:** Keep track of your potassium intake throughout the day, especially when consuming moderate-potassium foods, to ensure you stay within your recommended range.

By incorporating moderate-potassium foods in a controlled and balanced manner, you can enjoy a varied diet while managing your potassium levels effectively. Regular consultation with a healthcare provider or dietitian can further help tailor your diet to your specific needs.

3. Low Potassium Fruits and Vegetables

3.1 Fruits with Low Potassium Content

In managing a kidney-friendly diet, choosing fruits with low potassium content is crucial. These fruits provide essential vitamins, minerals, and fiber without significantly contributing to your daily potassium intake, making them safe and nutritious options for those with kidney disease.

Here's a list of fruits that are low in potassium, typically containing less than 200 mg per serving:

1. Apples

- **Potassium Content:** About 150 mg per medium apple.

- **Uses:** Apples are versatile and can be enjoyed fresh, baked, or as applesauce. They are great for snacking or adding to salads and desserts.

2. Berries

- **Strawberries:** About 120 mg per half-cup serving.
- **Blueberries:** Around 65 mg per half-cup serving.
- **Raspberries:** Approximately 95 mg per half-cup serving.
- **Uses:** Berries are low in potassium and rich in antioxidants. They can be eaten alone, added to cereals or yogurt, or used in smoothies and desserts.

3. Grapes

- **Potassium Content:** Around 150 mg per cup.
- **Uses:** Grapes are a hydrating and sweet option that can be eaten fresh, frozen for a cool treat, or used in salads and fruit dishes.

4. Pineapple

- **Potassium Content:** About 180 mg per cup.
- **Uses:** Fresh pineapple can be eaten on its own, added to fruit salads, or used in cooking to add a tropical flavor to dishes.

5. Pears

- **Potassium Content:** Approximately 180 mg per medium pear.
- **Uses:** Pears can be enjoyed fresh, canned, or baked. They're a delicious addition to salads, desserts, or as a simple snack.

6. Peaches

- **Potassium Content:** About 190 mg per medium peach.

- **Uses:** Peaches are a juicy, flavorful option that can be enjoyed fresh, canned (in water or juice), or used in desserts and smoothies.

7. Plums

- **Potassium Content:** Around 105 mg per small plum.
- **Uses:** Plums are low in potassium and can be eaten fresh, dried (as prunes, in moderation), or added to fruit salads and baked goods.

8. Cranberries

- **Potassium Content:** Roughly 20 mg per half-cup of fresh cranberries.
- **Uses:** Cranberries are very low in potassium and can be used in sauces, salads, or as a dried snack (note that dried cranberries are more concentrated in sugars).

9. Tangerines

- **Potassium Content:** About 150 mg per medium tangerine.
- **Uses:** Tangerines are a citrus fruit that can be eaten fresh, added to salads, or used as a flavorful garnish for various dishes.

10. Watermelon

- **Potassium Content:** Approximately 170 mg per cup of diced watermelon.
- **Uses:** Watermelon is hydrating and refreshing, perfect for eating on its own, in fruit salads, or as a cooling snack.

By incorporating these low-potassium fruits into your diet, you can enjoy a variety of sweet, nutritious options while effectively managing your potassium intake. Regular consumption of these fruits can help ensure that your diet remains both healthy and satisfying, supporting your overall well-being.

3.2 Vegetables with Low Potassium Content

Choosing vegetables with low potassium content is essential for those managing kidney disease. These vegetables provide vital nutrients without significantly increasing your potassium intake, making them safe and nutritious options to include in your diet. Here's a list of vegetables that are low in potassium, typically containing less than 200 mg per serving:

1. Lettuce

- **Potassium Content:** Approximately 20 mg per cup of shredded lettuce.
- **Uses:** Lettuce is a staple in salads, sandwiches, and wraps, offering a crisp texture and refreshing flavor.

2. Cucumbers

- **Potassium Content:** About 80 mg per half-cup of sliced cucumbers.
- **Uses:** Cucumbers are hydrating and can be enjoyed fresh in salads, as a snack, or as a garnish.

3. Bell Peppers

- **Potassium Content:** Around 130 mg per half-cup of sliced bell peppers.
- **Uses:** Bell peppers, particularly green ones, are versatile and can be added to salads, stir-fries, or eaten raw.

4. Green Beans

- **Potassium Content:** Approximately 90 mg per half-cup of cooked green beans.
- **Uses:** Green beans are a common side dish and can be added to casseroles, salads, or served on their own.

5. Onions

- **Potassium Content:** About 120 mg per half-cup of chopped onions.
- **Uses:** Onions add flavor to a variety of dishes, including salads, soups, and stir-fries.

6. Cabbage

- **Potassium Content:** Around 150 mg per cup of raw shredded cabbage.
- **Uses:** Cabbage can be used in salads, slaws, and as a component in various cooked dishes.

7. Zucchini

- **Potassium Content:** Approximately 170 mg per half-cup of sliced zucchini.
- **Uses:** Zucchini is a mild-tasting vegetable that can be added to salads, casseroles, or used as a pasta substitute.

8. Cauliflower

- **Potassium Content:** About 170 mg per half-cup of cooked cauliflower.
- **Uses:** Cauliflower is a versatile vegetable that can be included in salads, soups, or used as a low-carb substitute in various dishes.

9. Eggplant

- **Potassium Content:** Approximately 120 mg per half-cup of cooked eggplant.
- **Uses:** Eggplant is a hearty vegetable that can be grilled, baked, or added to stews and casseroles.

10. Radishes

- **Potassium Content:** Around 135 mg per half-cup of sliced radishes.
- **Uses:** Radishes add a peppery crunch to salads and can be eaten as a snack or garnish.

These low-potassium vegetables can be easily incorporated into your diet, providing essential nutrients while helping you manage your potassium intake. By choosing these vegetables, you can enjoy a wide variety of flavors and textures, all while supporting your kidney health.

3.3 Cooking Tips to Reduce Potassium in Fruits and Vegetables

For individuals with kidney disease, managing potassium intake is critical, and one effective way to reduce potassium content in fruits and vegetables is through specific cooking methods. These techniques can help make higher-potassium foods safer to consume by lowering their potassium levels.

Here are some cooking tips to help reduce potassium in fruits and vegetables:

1. Leaching

- **Method:** Leaching involves soaking vegetables in water to draw out some of the potassium. This method is particularly effective for starchy vegetables like potatoes, sweet potatoes, and carrots.
- **Steps:**

  - Peel and cut the vegetables into small, thin pieces.
  - Soak the vegetables in a large pot of water for at least 2 hours. Using a large amount of water relative to the amount of vegetables is key.
  - After soaking, rinse the vegetables under running water to remove any residual potassium.

- Cook the vegetables using a preferred method, such as boiling or steaming, to further reduce potassium.

2. Boiling

- **Method:** Boiling is one of the most effective ways to reduce potassium content in fruits and vegetables. The potassium leaches out of the food and into the water, which is then discarded.
- **Steps:**

  - Peel and cut the fruits or vegetables into small pieces.
  - Place them in a pot of water. Use a large amount of water to maximize potassium removal.
  - Boil the vegetables until tender. For fruits, boil for a shorter time to maintain texture.
  - Drain and discard the water immediately after boiling.

3. Double Boiling

- **Method:** Double boiling, or double-cooking, is a technique where the food is boiled in water, drained, and then boiled again in fresh water to further reduce potassium.
- **Steps:**

  - Peel and cut the fruits or vegetables into small pieces.
  - Boil the food in a large pot of water.
  - After the first boil, drain the water completely and replace it with fresh water.
  - Boil the food again until fully cooked, then drain and discard the water.

4. Blanching

- **Method:** Blanching involves briefly boiling fruits or vegetables and then plunging them into ice water to stop the cooking process. While blanching doesn't reduce potassium as much as boiling, it can still lower potassium levels, especially when followed by another cooking method.
- **Steps:**

    - Bring a pot of water to a boil.
    - Add the fruits or vegetables and boil for a short time (usually 2-3 minutes).
    - Immediately transfer the food to a bowl of ice water to stop the cooking process.
    - Drain the food and proceed with another cooking method if needed.

5. Steaming (with leaching)

- **Method:** Steaming is a gentle cooking method that helps preserve nutrients, but it can also be combined with leaching to reduce potassium content.
- **Steps:**

    - Soak the fruits or vegetables in water as described in the leaching process.
    - After soaking, drain the vegetables and place them in a steamer basket.
    - Steam the food over boiling water until tender.
    - Steaming after leaching can be particularly effective for vegetables like carrots and squash.

6. Peeling and Slicing

- **Method:** Potassium is often concentrated in the skin of fruits and vegetables. Peeling and slicing the food before cooking can help reduce its potassium content.
- **Steps:**

- Peel the skin off fruits and vegetables like potatoes, apples, and carrots.
- Slice the food into small, thin pieces to increase the surface area, allowing more potassium to leach out during cooking.
- Proceed with boiling, leaching, or another cooking method to further reduce potassium.

7. Avoiding Cooking in Small Amounts of Water

- **Method:** Cooking fruits and vegetables in small amounts of water or cooking them in their own juices can retain more potassium. Always use a large amount of water and discard the cooking liquid to ensure potassium is removed.
- **Steps:**

  - Cook the fruits or vegetables in a large pot with plenty of water.
  - Avoid using the cooking liquid in soups, gravies, or sauces, as it will contain potassium.

By incorporating these cooking tips into your food preparation routine, you can effectively reduce the potassium content in fruits and vegetables, making them safer for consumption within a kidney-friendly diet. These techniques allow you to enjoy a wider variety of foods while managing your potassium intake and supporting your overall health.

4. Low Potassium Protein Sources

4.1 Meat and Poultry

Meat and poultry are important sources of protein, iron, and other essential nutrients, making them a staple in many diets. However, for individuals with kidney disease, it's crucial to be mindful of the potassium content in these foods, as well as other factors that can impact kidney health, such as phosphorus and sodium levels. While meat and poultry typically contain moderate amounts of potassium, there are ways to incorporate these proteins into a kidney-friendly diet by carefully choosing cuts, portion sizes, and preparation methods.

1. Choosing Low-Potassium Cuts

- **White Meat (Poultry):** Chicken and turkey breast are generally lower in potassium compared to dark meat and other cuts. For example, a 3-ounce serving of skinless, boneless chicken breast contains around 220 mg of potassium, making it a safer choice when portioned appropriately.
- **Lean Cuts of Meat:** Lean cuts of meat, such as pork loin or beef sirloin, tend to be lower in potassium and fat compared to fattier cuts like ribs or chuck roast. A 3-ounce serving of pork loin contains approximately 300 mg of potassium.

2. Portion Control

- **Moderation is Key:** While meat and poultry can be part of a kidney-friendly diet, it's important to consume them in moderation. A typical serving size should be around 3 ounces (about the size of a deck of cards). This helps keep potassium intake within safe limits while still providing essential nutrients.
- **Balancing with Low-Potassium Foods:** Pairing meat or poultry with low-potassium vegetables, grains, and fruits can help create a balanced meal that supports kidney health.

3. Avoiding Processed Meats

- **Processed Meats:** Processed meats such as sausages, hot dogs, deli meats, and bacon often contain high levels of sodium, potassium additives, and phosphorus, which can be harmful to kidney health. It's best to avoid these or consume them only occasionally in very small amounts.

- **Fresh, Unprocessed Options:** Opt for fresh, unprocessed meats and poultry, as they are generally lower in additives that can increase the burden on the kidneys.

4. Cooking Methods

- **Grilling, Baking, or Broiling:** These cooking methods are ideal for meat and poultry, as they don't require adding extra sodium or potassium. They also allow excess fat to drain away, which can be beneficial for overall health.
- **Avoiding Salt and High-Potassium Marinades:** Use herbs, spices, and low-sodium seasonings to flavor your meat and poultry. Avoid using marinades or sauces that are high in potassium or sodium, such as soy sauce or certain barbecue sauces.

5. Monitoring Phosphorus Content

- **Phosphorus Concerns:** While focusing on potassium is essential, it's also important to monitor phosphorus intake, as high phosphorus levels can lead to bone and heart problems in people with kidney disease. Animal proteins, including meat and poultry, are often high in phosphorus, so it's important to consult with a dietitian to balance your diet appropriately.
- **Choosing Lower-Phosphorus Options:** Lean cuts of meat and poultry are generally lower in phosphorus. Also, opt for fresh cuts rather than processed ones to avoid added phosphorus.

Incorporating meat and poultry into a kidney-friendly diet requires careful selection and preparation. By choosing lean, unprocessed cuts, controlling portion sizes, and avoiding high-sodium or high-potassium additives, you can enjoy these protein-rich foods while supporting your kidney health. Always consult with a healthcare provider or dietitian to tailor your diet to your specific needs.

4.2 Seafood

Seafood is a rich source of high-quality protein, omega-3 fatty acids, and other essential nutrients that can be beneficial for overall health. However, for individuals with kidney disease, it's important to choose seafood options carefully, as some types are higher in potassium and phosphorus, which need to be managed within a kidney-friendly diet.

Here's a guide to selecting and preparing seafood that aligns with the dietary needs of kidney disease patients:

1. Choosing Lower Potassium Seafood

- **Fish with Lower Potassium Content:** Some fish are lower in potassium and can be safely included in a kidney-friendly diet when consumed in appropriate portions. Examples include:

  - **Cod:** A 3-ounce serving of cod contains about 240 mg of potassium, making it a relatively safe choice.
  - **Tilapia:** With approximately 280 mg of potassium per 3-ounce serving, tilapia is another good option.
  - **Sole and Flounder:** Both of these white fish varieties are low in potassium, with around 220 mg per 3-ounce serving.

- **Shellfish:** Shellfish like shrimp, crab, and scallops are generally lower in potassium compared to many types of fish. For example:

  - **Shrimp:** A 3-ounce serving of shrimp contains about 190 mg of potassium.
  - **Scallops:** Scallops contain around 270 mg of potassium per 3-ounce serving.

2. Managing Phosphorus Intake

- **Lower-Phosphorus Options:** While seafood is generally lower in potassium, it can be higher in phosphorus, which is also a concern for kidney disease patients. Opt for lower-phosphorus seafood such as:

  - **Salmon:** While salmon is slightly higher in potassium (around 380 mg per 3-ounce serving), it is rich in omega-3 fatty acids and has a moderate phosphorus content, making it a good option when consumed in moderation.
  - **Cod and Tilapia:** These fish not only have lower potassium levels but also contain moderate amounts of phosphorus, making them suitable choices.

- **Avoiding High-Phosphorus Seafood:** Certain seafood, such as sardines, mackerel, and anchovies, are higher in phosphorus and should be consumed sparingly or avoided, especially if phosphorus control is a priority in your diet.

3. Portion Control

- **Serving Size:** As with meat and poultry, it's important to keep seafood portions moderate to manage potassium and phosphorus intake. A 3-ounce serving (about the size of a deck of cards) is typically recommended.
- **Balancing Meals:** Pairing seafood with low-potassium vegetables or grains can help create a balanced, kidney-friendly meal.

4. Cooking Methods

- **Grilling, Baking, and Broiling:** These methods are ideal for preparing seafood, as they help retain the fish's natural flavors without the need for additional sodium or high-potassium ingredients.
- **Steaming and Poaching:** These gentle cooking methods are also excellent for preparing seafood, allowing you to enjoy the full nutritional benefits without adding unnecessary fats or sodium.

- **Avoiding High-Sodium Additives:** When preparing seafood, avoid using high-sodium marinades, sauces, or seasonings. Instead, opt for herbs, lemon juice, or low-sodium spices to enhance the flavor.

5. Omega-3 Fatty Acids

- **Heart Health Benefits:** Omega-3 fatty acids, found in fatty fish like salmon, mackerel, and sardines, are known for their heart health benefits. However, because these fish are higher in potassium and phosphorus, they should be consumed in moderation and as part of a balanced diet.
- **Supplements:** If you need to limit your intake of omega-3-rich fish due to potassium or phosphorus concerns, discuss with your healthcare provider whether omega-3 supplements might be an appropriate alternative.

6. Avoiding Processed Seafood

- **Canned and Smoked Seafood:** Processed seafood, such as canned or smoked fish, often contains high levels of sodium, phosphorus additives, and sometimes potassium. It's best to choose fresh or frozen seafood without added salts or preservatives to avoid these hidden sources of potassium and phosphorus.

By carefully selecting and preparing seafood, individuals with kidney disease can enjoy the nutritional benefits of these foods while managing their potassium and phosphorus intake. Consulting with a healthcare provider or dietitian can help tailor seafood choices to your specific dietary needs, ensuring a healthy and enjoyable diet.

4.3 Plant-Based Proteins

Plant-based proteins are an excellent alternative to animal proteins, offering a range of health benefits, including being lower in fat and calories. For individuals with kidney disease, choosing the right plant-based proteins is crucial, as some options can be higher in potassium and phosphorus. However, with careful selection and portion control, plant-based proteins can be a valuable part of a kidney-friendly diet.

1. Low-Potassium Plant-Based Proteins

- **Tofu:** Tofu is a versatile and low-potassium plant-based protein, with approximately 121 mg of potassium per half-cup serving. It can be used in a variety of dishes, from stir-fries to salads, providing a good source of protein without a significant potassium load.
- **Tempeh:** Tempeh, a fermented soybean product, contains about 260 mg of potassium per half-cup serving. While slightly higher in potassium than tofu, it is still a reasonable option when consumed in moderation.
- **Chickpeas (Garbanzo Beans):** Canned chickpeas have about 173 mg of potassium per half-cup serving when drained and rinsed. They can be used in salads, stews, or as a base for hummus.
- **Lentils:** Cooked lentils contain approximately 366 mg of potassium per half-cup serving, making them a higher-potassium option but still manageable in small portions.

2. Managing Phosphorus in Plant-Based Proteins

- **Lower-Phosphorus Options:** Some plant-based proteins, like lentils and beans, can be higher in phosphorus. It's important to manage portion sizes and balance these with other lower-phosphorus foods. Generally, tofu, edamame, and some types of beans, when portioned correctly, are good choices.

- **Phosphorus Absorption:** The phosphorus found in plant-based foods is typically in a form called phytate, which is less easily absorbed by the body compared to the phosphorus in animal proteins. This can be an advantage for individuals with kidney disease, as it allows for greater flexibility in including these foods in the diet.

3. Incorporating Whole Grains

- **Quinoa:** Quinoa is a complete protein, meaning it contains all nine essential amino acids. It has about 159 mg of potassium per half-cup cooked serving, making it a good option for those looking to increase their protein intake without excessive potassium.
- **Amaranth:** Amaranth is another whole grain that is high in protein and low in potassium, with around 116 mg of potassium per half-cup cooked serving.
- **Bulgur and Barley:** These grains are lower in potassium and can be excellent sources of protein and fiber. For example, cooked bulgur has approximately 62 mg of potassium per half-cup serving.

4. Nuts and Seeds: Moderation is Key

- **Almonds, Walnuts, and Flaxseeds:** These nuts and seeds are rich in healthy fats, protein, and fiber. However, they are also higher in potassium and phosphorus. For instance, a quarter-cup of almonds contains about 200 mg of potassium and 134 mg of phosphorus. Therefore, it's important to consume them in small amounts.
- **Chia Seeds:** Chia seeds are another high-protein, low-potassium option with around 44 mg of potassium per tablespoon. They can be added to smoothies, yogurts, or used to make chia pudding.

5. Legumes and Beans: High in Protein, Monitor Intake

- **Black Beans, Kidney Beans, and Pinto Beans:** These legumes are excellent plant-based protein sources but are higher in potassium, with black beans containing about 305 mg per half-cup serving. Consuming these in moderation and pairing them with low-potassium vegetables can help manage overall potassium intake.

- **Green Peas:** Green peas offer a lower-potassium alternative with about 88 mg of potassium per half-cup cooked serving. They can be included in salads, soups, or as a side dish.

6. Benefits of Plant-Based Proteins

- **Lower in Saturated Fat:** Plant-based proteins are generally lower in saturated fat compared to animal proteins, which can benefit heart health, a concern for many kidney disease patients.
- **High in Fiber:** Many plant-based proteins are high in fiber, which aids in digestion and helps regulate blood sugar levels. This is particularly important for kidney disease patients who may also be managing diabetes.

7. Cooking and Preparation Tips

- **Rinsing Canned Beans:** Rinsing canned beans under running water can help reduce their potassium and sodium content, making them safer for kidney patients to consume.
- **Soaking Dried Beans:** Soaking dried beans overnight and discarding the soaking water before cooking can help lower their potassium content.
- **Portion Control:** Even with plant-based proteins, portion control is essential to managing potassium and phosphorus intake. Pairing these proteins with low-potassium vegetables and grains can help create balanced meals.

Plant-based proteins offer a nutritious and often lower-fat alternative to animal proteins, making them a valuable part of a kidney-friendly diet. By carefully selecting low-potassium options, managing portion sizes, and preparing these foods in a way that minimizes potassium and phosphorus content, individuals with kidney disease can enjoy the benefits of plant-based proteins while supporting their kidney health.

5. Grains, Breads, and Cereals

5.1 Low Potassium Grains and Cereals

Grains and cereals are an essential part of a balanced diet, providing carbohydrates, fiber, vitamins, and minerals. For individuals with kidney disease, selecting low-potassium grains and cereals is crucial to maintaining healthy potassium levels while ensuring adequate nutrition. Fortunately, many grains and cereals are naturally low in potassium and can be safely incorporated into a kidney-friendly diet.

1. Rice

- **White Rice:** White rice is a staple grain that is low in potassium, making it an excellent choice for kidney disease patients. A half-cup serving of cooked white rice contains approximately 26 mg of potassium, which is minimal and safe for those monitoring their potassium intake.
- **Brown Rice:** While brown rice is more nutrient-dense than white rice, it is also higher in potassium, with around 86 mg per half-cup serving. If brown rice is preferred for its fiber content, it should be consumed in moderation and balanced with other low-potassium foods.

2. Pasta

- **Regular Pasta:** Regular white pasta is another low-potassium grain option, with about 30 mg of potassium per half-cup cooked serving. It is versatile and can be paired with various low-potassium vegetables and lean proteins to create a complete meal.
- **Whole Wheat Pasta:** Whole wheat pasta contains more fiber and nutrients than white pasta but is also higher in

potassium, with around 62 mg per half-cup serving. Like brown rice, it should be consumed in moderation.

3. Bread

- **White Bread:** White bread is generally low in potassium, with a slice containing about 30 mg of potassium. It can be a staple in a kidney-friendly diet when consumed in appropriate portions.
- **Whole Wheat Bread:** Whole wheat bread has more fiber and nutrients but also more potassium, with approximately 70 mg per slice. If whole wheat bread is preferred, it's important to monitor intake and adjust portions as needed.

4. Oats

- **Instant Oatmeal:** Instant oatmeal is a low-potassium breakfast option, with around 70 mg of potassium per half-cup cooked serving. It's quick to prepare and can be flavored with low-potassium fruits like blueberries or apples.
- **Rolled Oats:** Rolled oats are slightly higher in potassium, with about 105 mg per half-cup cooked serving. They are still a viable option but should be consumed in moderation.

5. Quinoa

- **Quinoa:** Quinoa is a complete protein grain that is lower in potassium than many other whole grains, with about 159 mg of potassium per half-cup cooked serving. It provides essential nutrients like protein, fiber, and magnesium, making it a nutritious choice for kidney patients when consumed in moderation.

6. Barley

- **Pearled Barley:** Pearled barley is a low-potassium grain with around 80 mg of potassium per half-cup cooked serving. It's high in fiber and can be used in soups, stews, or as a side dish.

- **Hulled Barley:** Hulled barley, while more nutritious, contains slightly more potassium. It should be portioned carefully if included in a kidney-friendly diet.

7. Corn and Cornmeal

- **Corn:** Corn is naturally low in potassium, with about 150 mg per half-cup serving. Corn-based products like tortillas and cornmeal are also low in potassium, making them good options for a kidney-friendly diet.
- **Polenta:** Polenta, a dish made from cornmeal, is low in potassium, with about 70 mg per half-cup cooked serving. It can be a versatile base for various meals.

8. Bulgur

- **Bulgur:** Bulgur is a whole grain that is lower in potassium than many other grains, with approximately 62 mg of potassium per half-cup cooked serving. It's high in fiber and can be used in salads, soups, and side dishes.

9. Couscous

- **Couscous:** Made from semolina wheat, couscous is a low-potassium grain with about 40 mg of potassium per half-cup cooked serving. It's quick to prepare and can be paired with various low-potassium ingredients for a balanced meal.

10. Breakfast Cereals

- **Low-Potassium Cereals:** Many breakfast cereals are low in potassium, especially those made from refined grains like cornflakes, puffed rice, and crisped rice. These cereals typically contain less than 50 mg of potassium per serving, making them a safe choice for a kidney-friendly diet.
- **Avoiding High-Potassium Additives:** When selecting cereals, avoid those with added nuts, seeds, or dried fruits,

as these can increase the potassium content. Opt for plain cereals and add fresh, low-potassium fruits if desired.

By choosing the right grains and cereals, individuals with kidney disease can enjoy a variety of satisfying and nutritious foods while managing their potassium intake. These low-potassium options provide the energy and nutrients needed to support overall health, making them a valuable component of a kidney-friendly diet.

5.2 Choosing the Right Bread Products

Bread is a dietary staple for many people, but for those with kidney disease, it's important to choose the right bread products to manage potassium, sodium, and phosphorus intake. While bread can be low in potassium, different types of bread vary in their nutritional content, so careful selection is key to maintaining a kidney-friendly diet.

1. Understanding Potassium Content in Bread

- **White Bread:** White bread is typically lower in potassium than whole wheat or multigrain bread, with around 25-30 mg of potassium per slice. This makes it a safe choice for those needing to limit their potassium intake. The refining process removes much of the potassium content found in whole grains, resulting in a lower potassium product.
- **Whole Wheat Bread:** Whole wheat bread contains more potassium, with about 70 mg per slice, due to the inclusion of the entire wheat grain. While whole wheat bread is more nutritious and higher in fiber, it's important to consume it in moderation if potassium intake needs to be limited.
- **Multigrain Bread:** Multigrain bread, made from a variety of grains and seeds, can vary widely in potassium content depending on the ingredients used. Some multigrain breads may contain nuts or seeds, which are higher in potassium, so it's essential to check the nutrition label.

2. Managing Phosphorus in Bread

- **Phosphorus Additives:** Some bread products contain added phosphorus, often in the form of preservatives or dough conditioners. These additives can significantly increase the phosphorus content of the bread. It's important to read labels and avoid breads that list phosphorus additives, such as calcium phosphate or phosphoric acid.
- **Whole Grain Bread:** Whole grain breads naturally contain more phosphorus than refined breads. While the phosphorus in plant-based foods is not as easily absorbed by the body as that in animal products, those with advanced kidney disease may still need to monitor their intake. Consuming whole grain bread in moderation and balancing it with lower-phosphorus foods can help manage overall phosphorus levels.

3. Sodium Content in Bread

- **Low-Sodium Bread:** Bread can be a hidden source of sodium, which is a concern for kidney disease patients. Low-sodium bread options are available and should be chosen whenever possible, as they typically contain less than 140 mg of sodium per slice. Reducing sodium intake is important to help control blood pressure and fluid balance, both of which are crucial for kidney health.
- **Regular Bread:** Standard bread products can contain anywhere from 150-250 mg of sodium per slice, so it's important to be mindful of portion sizes. Limiting the number of slices or opting for low-sodium varieties can help keep sodium intake in check.

4. Specialty Bread Products

- **Gluten-Free Bread:** For those with gluten intolerance or celiac disease, gluten-free bread is a necessary alternative. Many gluten-free breads are made from rice, corn, or potato flours, which are low in potassium. However, it's important to check the label for added potassium chloride, which can increase the potassium content.

- **Sourdough Bread:** Sourdough bread is often lower in sodium than regular bread and has a unique tangy flavor due to the fermentation process. It typically has around 40-60 mg of potassium per slice, making it a reasonable choice for those monitoring their potassium intake.

5. Serving Sizes and Bread Choices

- **Portion Control:** Even with lower-potassium and low-sodium bread options, portion control is crucial. Sticking to one or two slices per meal can help manage overall potassium, phosphorus, and sodium intake. Pairing bread with low-potassium spreads or toppings, such as butter, cream cheese, or jam, can further help in maintaining a kidney-friendly diet.
- **Bread as a Meal Component:** Incorporating bread as part of a balanced meal with low-potassium vegetables, lean proteins, or plant-based proteins can help ensure that overall dietary intake is aligned with kidney health goals.

6. Reading Nutrition Labels

- **Key Ingredients to Watch For:** When selecting bread products, always read the nutrition labels carefully. Look for breads with minimal sodium, low potassium, and no added phosphorus. Ingredients like potassium chloride, calcium phosphate, or other phosphate additives should be avoided if you are trying to manage phosphorus and potassium intake.
- **Choosing Simple, Less Processed Breads:** Opting for simpler, less processed bread products with fewer ingredients is generally a good strategy. The fewer additives, the easier it is to control potassium and phosphorus intake.

By choosing the right bread products and being mindful of portion sizes, individuals with kidney disease can enjoy bread as part of a healthy, balanced diet. Low-potassium, low-sodium bread options provide a versatile and satisfying foundation for meals while supporting the dietary restrictions necessary for kidney health.

5.3 Low Potassium Snacks

Snacking is an essential part of a balanced diet, offering the energy needed between meals to keep you going throughout the day. For individuals with kidney disease, it's important to choose snacks that are low in potassium to avoid putting extra strain on the kidneys. Fortunately, there are plenty of tasty, low-potassium snacks that can satisfy cravings while supporting kidney health.

1. Fresh Fruits

- **Apples:** Apples are a kidney-friendly fruit, with about 130 mg of potassium in a medium-sized apple. They are versatile and can be eaten fresh, sliced with peanut butter, or added to salads.
- **Berries:** Strawberries, blueberries, and raspberries are all low in potassium, with less than 150 mg per half-cup serving. These berries can be enjoyed on their own, mixed into yogurt, or blended into smoothies.
- **Grapes:** A cup of grapes contains about 288 mg of potassium, making them a good choice for a low-potassium snack. They are easy to pack and can be eaten fresh or frozen for a refreshing treat.

2. Vegetables

- **Cucumber Slices:** Cucumbers are very low in potassium, with only about 80 mg per cup of sliced cucumber. They make a crisp, hydrating snack and can be paired with low-potassium dips like hummus or ranch dressing.
- **Carrot Sticks:** Carrots are another great low-potassium option, containing about 195 mg of potassium per half-cup serving of raw carrot sticks. They are crunchy and can be

dipped in hummus or a low-potassium dressing for added flavor.
- **Celery Sticks:** Celery is extremely low in potassium, with just 88 mg per cup of chopped celery. It's a perfect snack when paired with peanut butter or a small amount of cream cheese.

3. Crackers and Rice Cakes

- **Unsalted Crackers:** Unsalted or low-sodium crackers are a good snack choice for those watching their potassium and sodium intake. These crackers typically contain around 25-50 mg of potassium per serving and can be paired with low-potassium toppings like cream cheese or cucumber slices.
- **Rice Cakes:** Plain rice cakes are low in potassium, with about 35 mg per cake. They are light and crunchy, making them an ideal base for a variety of toppings, such as sliced apples, peanut butter, or a sprinkle of cinnamon.

4. Popcorn

- **Air-Popped Popcorn:** Air-popped popcorn is a low-potassium, low-calorie snack option, with around 30 mg of potassium per cup. It's also high in fiber, making it a filling snack. To keep it kidney-friendly, avoid adding too much salt or butter; instead, try seasoning it with herbs or a sprinkle of garlic powder.

5. Low-Potassium Dips

- **Hummus:** Traditional hummus made from chickpeas contains about 99 mg of potassium per tablespoon. While it does contain some potassium, small portions paired with low-potassium vegetables like cucumber or carrot sticks make it a viable snack option.
- **Cream Cheese:** Cream cheese is naturally low in potassium, with around 20 mg per tablespoon. It can be spread on crackers, rice cakes, or used as a dip for fresh vegetables.

- **Greek Yogurt:** Plain Greek yogurt is a low-potassium snack with around 150 mg of potassium per half-cup serving. It can be enjoyed on its own, with fresh berries, or as a base for homemade dips.

6. Nuts and Seeds

- **Unsalted Peanuts:** Peanuts are lower in potassium compared to other nuts, with about 200 mg of potassium per quarter-cup serving. While they should be consumed in moderation, they provide protein and healthy fats that make for a satisfying snack.
- **Pumpkin Seeds:** Pumpkin seeds are relatively low in potassium, with about 226 mg per quarter-cup serving. Choose unsalted varieties and enjoy them in small portions.

7. Low-Potassium Sweet Treats

- **Rice Pudding:** Rice pudding made with white rice and milk is a low-potassium sweet treat, especially when prepared with a small amount of sugar and topped with cinnamon.
- **Gelatin Desserts:** Gelatin-based desserts like Jell-O are low in potassium, with only about 1 mg per serving. They can be flavored with fruit juice and offer a refreshing, low-potassium snack.
- **Marshmallows:** Marshmallows are a fun, low-potassium treat, with less than 2 mg of potassium per regular-sized marshmallow. They can be enjoyed on their own or added to a low-potassium hot chocolate.

8. Dairy Alternatives

- **Almond Milk:** Unsweetened almond milk is low in potassium, with about 150 mg per cup. It can be used as a base for smoothies or enjoyed on its own as a light snack.
- **Coconut Yogurt:** Coconut yogurt is a dairy-free alternative that is lower in potassium than traditional

yogurt. It can be enjoyed with low-potassium fruits or on its own as a snack.

9. Small Portions of Sweets

- **Gummy Candies:** Most gummy candies are low in potassium and can be enjoyed occasionally. Just be mindful of sugar content and consume in moderation.
- **Hard Candies:** Hard candies like peppermints or fruit-flavored drops are low in potassium and can be a quick, sweet snack when you need a little treat.

By selecting these low-potassium snacks, individuals with kidney disease can enjoy a variety of delicious options throughout the day without compromising their dietary needs. These snacks not only help manage potassium levels but also provide the necessary energy and nutrients to maintain overall health.

6. Dairy and Dairy Alternatives

6.1 Low Potassium Dairy Products

Dairy products are a rich source of calcium, protein, and other essential nutrients, but they can also be high in potassium, which poses a challenge for individuals with kidney disease. However, there are several low-potassium dairy options that can be safely included in a kidney-friendly diet. These options allow for the enjoyment of dairy's benefits while keeping potassium levels in check.

1. Milk Alternatives

- **Almond Milk:** Unsweetened almond milk is one of the lowest-potassium milk alternatives, with about 150 mg of potassium per cup. It's a versatile substitute for cow's milk and can be used in cereal, smoothies, coffee, and baking. It also has the added benefit of being lower in calories.

- **Rice Milk:** Rice milk is another low-potassium option, containing approximately 60 mg of potassium per cup. It has a mild flavor and can be used similarly to almond milk. Opt for the unsweetened version to avoid excess sugar intake.
- **Coconut Milk:** Coconut milk (from cartons, not canned) typically contains around 50-60 mg of potassium per cup. It's a creamy alternative to cow's milk and is especially good in smoothies, desserts, or as a coffee creamer.

2. Cheese

- **Cream Cheese:** Cream cheese is a low-potassium spread with about 20 mg of potassium per tablespoon. It can be used on bagels, crackers, or as a base for dips and is also relatively low in sodium when choosing plain varieties.
- **Cottage Cheese (in Moderation):** While cottage cheese has more potassium than other cheese options, with around 200 mg per half-cup, it is still lower than many other dairy products. It can be included in small portions as part of a balanced diet, particularly when paired with low-potassium fruits like pineapple or berries.
- **Ricotta Cheese:** Ricotta cheese is another lower-potassium option, with about 150 mg per half-cup serving. It's creamy and mild, making it a great addition to dishes like lasagna, stuffed shells, or even as a spread on toast.

3. Yogurt

- **Greek Yogurt:** Plain Greek yogurt contains about 150 mg of potassium per half-cup serving. While it does contain potassium, it's lower than many other dairy products and can be a good option when eaten in moderation. It's high in protein and can be paired with low-potassium fruits or honey for added flavor.
- **Coconut Yogurt:** Coconut yogurt, made from coconut milk, is lower in potassium compared to traditional yogurt. It typically contains around 100-150 mg of potassium per

half-cup serving, depending on the brand. It's a good alternative for those who prefer a dairy-free option.

4. Butter and Margarine

- **Butter:** Butter is low in potassium, with only about 3 mg per tablespoon. It's a safe option for spreading on bread, cooking, or baking. While butter is high in saturated fat, it can be used in moderation as part of a balanced diet.
- **Margarine:** Many margarine products are low in potassium, but it's important to choose varieties that are low in trans fats and sodium. Stick margarine often contains higher trans fats, so soft or tub margarine is generally a better choice.

5. Low Potassium Ice Cream and Desserts

- **Vanilla Ice Cream:** Regular vanilla ice cream typically contains around 150-170 mg of potassium per half-cup serving. While it's not the lowest-potassium option, it can be enjoyed occasionally in small portions. Some brands offer lower potassium content, so checking the label is key.
- **Sherbet:** Sherbet is generally lower in potassium than ice cream, with about 60 mg per half-cup serving. It's a refreshing dessert alternative with a fruity flavor, and it's lower in fat and calories as well.
- **Whipped Topping:** Whipped topping, either from a can or homemade, is low in potassium, with around 1-2 mg per tablespoon. It can be used to top desserts like pies or as a light addition to fruits.

6. Specialty Low-Potassium Dairy Products

- **Low-Potassium Cheese:** Some specialty cheeses are made specifically for people with kidney disease, with reduced potassium and phosphorus levels. These can be a good option for those who want to enjoy cheese without worrying about potassium intake.
- **Lactose-Free Milk:** Lactose-free milk is similar in potassium content to regular cow's milk but is easier to

digest for those with lactose intolerance. Some brands offer lower-potassium versions, so it's worth exploring different products to find the best fit.

By choosing these low-potassium dairy products, individuals with kidney disease can continue to enjoy the nutritional benefits of dairy while managing their potassium intake. These options provide a balance between maintaining kidney health and enjoying a varied, satisfying diet.

6.2 Plant-Based Milk and Alternatives

For individuals with kidney disease, managing potassium levels is crucial, and plant-based milk and alternatives can provide a nutritious, low-potassium option. These dairy-free alternatives are not only lower in potassium than cow's milk but also cater to those with lactose intolerance, dairy allergies, or those following a plant-based diet. Here's a closer look at some popular plant-based milk options and how they can fit into a kidney-friendly diet.

1. Almond Milk

- **Low Potassium Content:** Unsweetened almond milk is one of the lowest-potassium milk alternatives, with approximately 150 mg of potassium per cup. This makes it an excellent choice for individuals looking to manage their potassium intake. It's also low in calories, with around 30-40 calories per cup, depending on the brand.
- **Versatility:** Almond milk has a light, nutty flavor that works well in a variety of dishes. It can be used in cereal, smoothies, coffee, and baking. It's also available in sweetened, unsweetened, and flavored varieties, though the unsweetened version is recommended for those monitoring sugar intake.

2. Rice Milk

- **Very Low Potassium:** Rice milk is another kidney-friendly option, with about 60 mg of potassium per cup. It's one of the lowest in potassium among plant-based milks, making it a safe choice for those with kidney disease.
- **Mild Flavor:** Rice milk has a mild, slightly sweet flavor and a thin consistency. It's a great option for drinking on its own or using in recipes that require a light milk substitute. Like almond milk, it's available in sweetened and unsweetened versions.

3. Coconut Milk

- **Moderate Potassium Content:** Carton coconut milk contains around 50-60 mg of potassium per cup, making it a suitable option for those needing to limit their potassium intake. Canned coconut milk, on the other hand, is much higher in potassium and should be used sparingly.
- **Creamy Texture:** Coconut milk has a creamy texture and a distinct, slightly sweet coconut flavor. It's particularly popular in smoothies, coffee, and baking. Coconut milk is also low in calories and can be found in both sweetened and unsweetened forms.

4. Oat Milk

- **Higher Potassium, Use with Caution:** Oat milk contains around 150-200 mg of potassium per cup, depending on the brand. While it's higher in potassium than almond, rice, or coconut milk, it can still be included in a kidney-friendly diet if consumed in moderation.
- **Rich and Creamy:** Oat milk has a rich, creamy texture that makes it a popular choice for coffee, lattes, and baking. It's naturally sweet and is often fortified with vitamins and minerals, including calcium and vitamin D, making it a nutritious choice.

5. Soy Milk

- **Moderate to High Potassium:** Soy milk has around 200-300 mg of potassium per cup, depending on the brand and whether it's fortified. Because of its higher potassium content, soy milk should be used with caution and in smaller amounts by those with kidney disease.
- **Protein-Rich:** Soy milk is high in protein, similar to cow's milk, and has a slightly thicker texture. It's a good source of plant-based protein and is often fortified with calcium and vitamins. For those who prefer soy milk, choosing an unsweetened variety can help control sugar intake.

6. Hemp Milk

- **Moderate Potassium Content:** Hemp milk contains around 100-200 mg of potassium per cup. It's relatively low in potassium compared to cow's milk but higher than some other plant-based options.
- **Nutty Flavor:** Hemp milk has a nutty flavor and a creamy texture, making it suitable for drinking on its own, in coffee, or in smoothies. It's also rich in omega-3 and omega-6 fatty acids, which are beneficial for heart health.

7. Pea Protein Milk

- **Moderate Potassium:** Pea protein milk, made from yellow peas, contains around 150-200 mg of potassium per cup. Like oat milk, it's higher in potassium but can be consumed in moderation.
- **High Protein Content:** Pea protein milk is similar to soy milk in terms of protein content, making it a good option for those needing more protein in their diet. It's also creamy and has a mild flavor that works well in various recipes.

8. Choosing the Right Plant-Based Milk

- **Reading Labels:** It's important to check the labels when selecting plant-based milk, as potassium content can vary between brands and even between different products from

the same brand. Look for options with the lowest potassium content and no added potassium chloride or other potassium-based additives.
- **Unsweetened Varieties:** Whenever possible, opt for unsweetened versions of plant-based milk to avoid added sugars, which can contribute to other health issues. Sweetened varieties can contain added sugars that are unnecessary and can increase calorie intake.

9. Using Plant-Based Milk in a Kidney-Friendly Diet

- **Portion Control:** Even with low-potassium plant-based milks, portion control is essential. Stick to one cup per serving and balance it with other low-potassium foods throughout the day.
- **Incorporating Variety:** Incorporating a variety of plant-based milks into your diet can help provide a range of nutrients while managing potassium levels. Try rotating between almond, rice, and coconut milk to keep your diet diverse and interesting.

Plant-based milk and alternatives offer a kidney-friendly way to enjoy the benefits of milk without the high potassium content found in cow's milk. By choosing low-potassium options and monitoring portion sizes, individuals with kidney disease can continue to enjoy milk in their diet while supporting their overall health.

7. Drinks and Beverages

7.1 Low Potassium Beverages

For individuals managing kidney disease, choosing the right beverages is crucial to controlling potassium intake and maintaining overall health. Many popular drinks can be high in potassium, so it's important to select options that are lower in potassium while still providing hydration and enjoyment. Here's a guide to low-potassium beverages that can fit well into a kidney-friendly diet.

1. Water

- **Potassium Content:** Water is naturally free of potassium, making it the best choice for hydration. It helps maintain fluid balance and supports overall kidney function without adding to potassium intake.
- **Variety:** Plain water can be enhanced with a splash of lemon or lime for added flavor without significantly increasing potassium levels. Infused water with cucumber, mint, or berries can also be a refreshing, low-potassium alternative.

2. Herbal Teas

- **Potassium Content:** Most herbal teas are low in potassium, typically containing less than 5 mg of potassium per serving. They offer a variety of flavors and can be enjoyed hot or iced.
- **Varieties:** Popular herbal teas include chamomile, peppermint, ginger, and rooibos. These teas are naturally caffeine-free and can be a soothing option for relaxation or a warm drink before bed.

3. Clear Broths

- **Potassium Content:** Clear broths, such as chicken, beef, or vegetable broth, are generally low in potassium when prepared without added salt or high-potassium vegetables. A cup of clear broth typically contains around 200-300 mg of potassium, but this can vary based on preparation.
- **Uses:** Clear broths can be consumed as a light snack or used as a base for soups and stews. Opt for low-sodium versions or homemade broths to control both potassium and sodium levels.

4. Lemonade

- **Potassium Content:** Lemonade made from fresh lemon juice and water is relatively low in potassium, with around 10-20 mg of potassium per cup. It's a refreshing option, especially when served chilled.
- **Preparation:** To keep lemonade kidney-friendly, avoid adding excessive amounts of sugar or potassium-based sweeteners. Use fresh lemon juice and dilute with plenty of water.

5. Cranberry Juice

- **Potassium Content:** Unsweetened cranberry juice typically contains around 150-200 mg of potassium per cup. While not the lowest in potassium, it is often lower than other fruit juices.
- **Consumption:** Drinking cranberry juice in moderation can provide a flavorful alternative to plain water. Opt for no-added-sugar varieties to reduce overall sugar intake.

6. Apple Juice

- **Potassium Content:** Apple juice contains about 200-250 mg of potassium per cup. While it's higher in potassium than some other beverages, it can still be included in a kidney-friendly diet when consumed in limited quantities.
- **Choice:** Choose 100% pure apple juice with no added sugars or potassium-based additives. Diluting apple juice with water can help reduce potassium intake while still providing some flavor.

7. Low-Potassium Smoothies

- **Potassium Content:** Smoothies made with low-potassium fruits, such as berries or apples, and low-potassium milk alternatives like almond milk or rice milk, can be a nutritious option. The potassium content will depend on the ingredients used.

- **Recipe Suggestions:** Combine unsweetened almond milk with a small amount of berries and a handful of ice for a low-potassium smoothie. Avoid high-potassium fruits like bananas and oranges to keep the potassium content low.

8. Sparkling Water

- **Potassium Content:** Plain sparkling water or seltzer water is typically low in potassium, similar to still water. It can be a great option for those who enjoy fizzy beverages.
- **Flavored Varieties:** Look for sparkling waters that are naturally flavored without added sugars or potassium-based additives. Adding a splash of fruit juice or a slice of lemon can enhance flavor without significantly affecting potassium levels.

9. Decaffeinated Coffee

- **Potassium Content:** Decaffeinated coffee contains less potassium than regular coffee, with about 100-150 mg of potassium per cup. While it's still important to monitor intake, decaffeinated coffee can be included in a low-potassium diet.
- **Preparation:** Opt for black decaffeinated coffee or use a low-potassium milk alternative to avoid adding excess potassium. Avoid adding high-potassium ingredients like chocolate or nuts.

10. Non-Dairy Creamers

- **Potassium Content:** Non-dairy creamers, particularly those made from almond or coconut milk, can be lower in potassium compared to traditional creamers. Check labels to ensure they meet potassium guidelines.
- **Usage:** Non-dairy creamers can be used in coffee or tea. Choose unsweetened versions to avoid added sugars and select products with lower potassium content.

By incorporating these low-potassium beverages into your daily routine, you can stay hydrated and enjoy a variety of drinks while managing your potassium intake. Always check labels and ingredients to ensure that the beverages you choose fit within your dietary restrictions and support your kidney health.

7.2 Beverages to Limit or Avoid

For individuals with kidney disease, carefully managing potassium intake is essential, and this extends to beverage choices. Certain drinks can be high in potassium, sodium, or other substances that may exacerbate kidney issues or overall health. Here's a guide to beverages that should be limited or avoided to maintain a kidney-friendly diet.

1. Regular Coffee

- **Potassium Content:** Regular coffee contains about 300-400 mg of potassium per cup. While it provides a stimulating effect, its high potassium content can contribute to excessive potassium intake, especially if consumed in large amounts.
- **Alternative:** Opt for decaffeinated coffee, which generally contains less potassium, or choose low-potassium beverages like herbal teas.

2. Orange Juice

- **Potassium Content:** Orange juice is high in potassium, with approximately 450-500 mg per cup. This makes it a less suitable choice for those needing to monitor their potassium intake.
- **Alternative:** Consider low-potassium fruit juices like cranberry or apple juice, and consume them in moderation.

3. Tomato Juice

- **Potassium Content:** Tomato juice is rich in potassium, with around 450-500 mg per cup. Its high potassium content can be problematic for individuals with kidney disease.
- **Alternative:** Opt for low-potassium vegetable juices or make your own broth-based drinks with controlled potassium levels.

4. Sports Drinks

- **Potassium Content:** Many sports drinks contain high levels of potassium, often around 200-250 mg per 12-ounce serving. They are designed to replenish electrolytes but can contribute to high potassium levels if consumed frequently.
- **Alternative:** Stick to plain water or low-potassium beverages for hydration, especially if you're not engaging in intense physical activity.

5. Energy Drinks

- **Potassium Content:** Energy drinks can contain high levels of potassium and other stimulants that may not be kidney-friendly. Potassium content varies but can be substantial.
- **Alternative:** Choose low-potassium beverages or herbal teas to avoid excess potassium and stimulants.

6. Milk (Cow's Milk)

- **Potassium Content:** Cow's milk contains about 300-400 mg of potassium per cup. While it is a good source of calcium and protein, it's high in potassium for those on a restricted diet.
- **Alternative:** Opt for plant-based milk alternatives with lower potassium content, such as almond or rice milk.

7. Alcoholic Beverages

- **Potassium Content:** While alcohol itself doesn't contain high levels of potassium, many mixed drinks and cocktails can be high in potassium due to their ingredients, such as fruit juices and syrups.
- **Alternative:** If you choose to drink alcohol, do so in moderation and be aware of the mixers used. Plain spirits like vodka or gin, consumed with low-potassium mixers, may be a better choice.

8. High-Sugar Fruit Juices

- **Potassium Content:** Fruit juices that are high in sugar, like grape or banana juice, can be high in potassium as well. They can contribute to overall potassium and sugar intake, which is a concern for kidney health.
- **Alternative:** Choose 100% juice with lower potassium content and drink it in moderation. Consider diluting with water to lower the overall potassium and sugar content.

9. Canned or Bottled Beverages with Added Potassium

- **Potassium Content:** Some canned or bottled beverages, including certain fruit-flavored drinks and enhanced waters, have added potassium for nutritional benefits. These should be avoided or consumed with caution.
- **Alternative:** Check labels for potassium content and opt for beverages without added potassium. Plain water or low-potassium alternatives are safer choices.

10. Highly Sweetened Beverages

- **Potassium Content:** Highly sweetened beverages like sodas and sugary drinks may not always be high in potassium, but they can contribute to overall health issues like diabetes and hypertension, which can impact kidney health.
- **Alternative:** Opt for beverages that are low in sugar and potassium, such as plain water, herbal teas, or diluted fruit juices.

11. Herbal Teas with High Potassium Content

- **Potassium Content:** While many herbal teas are low in potassium, some specialty herbal teas might contain higher levels depending on their ingredients.
- **Alternative:** Stick to well-known low-potassium herbal teas such as chamomile, peppermint, or rooibos.

By limiting or avoiding these high-potassium or problematic beverages, you can better manage your potassium intake and support kidney health. Always check labels and choose beverages that fit within your dietary guidelines to maintain overall well-being.

8. Seasonings, Herbs, and Condiments

8.1 Low Potassium Herbs and Spices

Herbs and spices are essential for adding flavor and variety to meals without adding extra sodium or calories. For individuals with kidney disease, choosing low-potassium herbs and spices can enhance the taste of food while helping to manage potassium intake. Here's a guide to low-potassium herbs and spices that can be safely used in a kidney-friendly diet.

1. Basil

- **Potassium Content:** Fresh basil contains approximately 30 mg of potassium per tablespoon, while dried basil has about 70 mg per tablespoon. It's a versatile herb that adds a fragrant, slightly sweet flavor to dishes.
- **Uses:** Basil is commonly used in Italian cuisine, in dishes such as pasta sauces, pesto, and salads. It pairs well with tomatoes, garlic, and olive oil.

2. Chives

- **Potassium Content:** Chives are very low in potassium, with about 10 mg per tablespoon of fresh chives. They provide a mild onion flavor that can brighten up a variety of dishes.
- **Uses:** Chives are great for garnishing soups, salads, and baked potatoes. They can also be added to omelets and dips for an extra burst of flavor.

3. Dill

- **Potassium Content:** Fresh dill contains around 50 mg of potassium per tablespoon. Dill adds a light, tangy flavor that complements fish, potatoes, and salads.
- **Uses:** Dill is commonly used in pickling, and its fresh leaves can be added to fish dishes, dressings, and vegetable dishes.

4. Parsley

- **Potassium Content:** Fresh parsley contains about 30 mg of potassium per tablespoon. It is a mild herb that enhances the flavor of many dishes without overwhelming other ingredients.
- **Uses:** Parsley is used as a garnish or in recipes like tabbouleh, soups, and sauces. It can also be blended into pesto or used in marinades.

5. Rosemary

- **Potassium Content:** Rosemary contains approximately 10 mg of potassium per teaspoon of dried herb. It has a strong, woody flavor that pairs well with roasted meats and vegetables.
- **Uses:** Rosemary is often used in roasting, grilling, and braising. It complements dishes such as roasted chicken, potatoes, and lamb.

6. Sage

- **Potassium Content:** Sage is low in potassium, with around 10 mg per teaspoon of dried sage. It offers a robust, earthy flavor that can enhance a variety of dishes.
- **Uses:** Sage is commonly used in stuffing, sausage dishes, and with poultry. It's also a key ingredient in traditional Thanksgiving recipes.

7. Thyme

- **Potassium Content:** Thyme has about 20 mg of potassium per teaspoon of dried herb. It provides a subtle, earthy flavor that works well in a variety of savory dishes.
- **Uses:** Thyme is versatile and can be used in soups, stews, marinades, and as a seasoning for meats and vegetables.

8. Turmeric

- **Potassium Content:** Turmeric has approximately 200 mg of potassium per teaspoon. Although slightly higher in potassium than some other spices, it can be used in moderation.
- **Uses:** Turmeric is known for its bright yellow color and earthy flavor. It's commonly used in curry powders, rice dishes, and soups.

9. Bay Leaves

- **Potassium Content:** Bay leaves are low in potassium, with around 10 mg per leaf. They are used primarily for flavoring and are typically removed before serving.
- **Uses:** Bay leaves are used in soups, stews, and braises to add a subtle, aromatic flavor. They should be removed from dishes before eating.

10. Cumin

- **Potassium Content:** Cumin contains about 20 mg of potassium per teaspoon. It adds a warm, earthy flavor to dishes.

- **Uses:** Cumin is used in a variety of cuisines, including Mexican, Indian, and Middle Eastern. It's commonly used in chili, curries, and spice blends.

11. Coriander

- **Potassium Content:** Ground coriander has about 10 mg of potassium per teaspoon. It offers a citrusy, slightly sweet flavor.
- **Uses:** Coriander is used in spice blends, soups, and stews. It's also an ingredient in many Mexican and Indian dishes.

12. Ginger

- **Potassium Content:** Fresh ginger contains approximately 20 mg of potassium per tablespoon. It adds a spicy, warm flavor to dishes.
- **Uses:** Ginger is used in both sweet and savory dishes, including stir-fries, marinades, and desserts. It's also a key ingredient in many Asian cuisines.

13. Cinnamon

- **Potassium Content:** Cinnamon contains about 30 mg of potassium per teaspoon. It provides a sweet, warm flavor that can enhance both savory and sweet dishes.
- **Uses:** Cinnamon is commonly used in baking, oatmeal, and spice blends. It's also used to flavor beverages like hot apple cider.

By incorporating these low-potassium herbs and spices into your diet, you can enhance the flavor of your meals without compromising your potassium restrictions. Using a variety of herbs and spices can help keep meals interesting and satisfying while adhering to dietary guidelines.

8.2 Safe Condiments and Sauces

Condiments and sauces are often used to enhance the flavor of meals, but many can be high in potassium, sodium, or other ingredients that may not be ideal for individuals with kidney disease. Choosing the right condiments and sauces can help manage potassium intake while still allowing you to enjoy flavorful dishes. Here's a guide to safe condiments and sauces that are generally low in potassium and can be included in a kidney-friendly diet.

1. Olive Oil

- **Potassium Content:** Olive oil is very low in potassium, with negligible amounts per serving. It is also a good source of healthy fats.
- **Uses:** Olive oil can be used as a base for salad dressings, a cooking oil, or a drizzle over vegetables and grains. It adds a rich flavor without adding potassium.

2. Balsamic Vinegar

- **Potassium Content:** Balsamic vinegar contains minimal potassium, about 10 mg per tablespoon. It is a great way to add tangy flavor to dishes.
- **Uses:** Balsamic vinegar can be used in salad dressings, marinades, and as a finishing touch on vegetables and meats.

3. Lemon Juice

- **Potassium Content:** Lemon juice is low in potassium, with about 10 mg per tablespoon. It adds a bright, acidic flavor to dishes.
- **Uses:** Lemon juice can be used in dressings, marinades, and to brighten the flavor of seafood, chicken, and vegetables.

4. Mustard

- **Potassium Content:** Most mustards are low in potassium, with about 5-10 mg per teaspoon. It adds a tangy, sharp flavor to foods.
- **Uses:** Mustard can be used in sandwiches, dressings, and as a flavoring for meats. Opt for varieties without added potassium-based ingredients.

5. Soy Sauce (Low Sodium)

- **Potassium Content:** Low-sodium soy sauce contains about 200-300 mg of potassium per tablespoon. While not as low in potassium as some other condiments, it can be used sparingly.
- **Uses:** Low-sodium soy sauce can be used in small amounts for flavoring stir-fries, sauces, and marinades.

6. Salsa

- **Potassium Content:** Fresh salsa made with tomatoes, onions, and herbs is generally lower in potassium than other tomato-based sauces, with about 150-200 mg per half-cup serving. Check labels for sodium content.
- **Uses:** Salsa can be used as a dip, topping for meats, or mixed into dishes like salads and rice. Opt for varieties with minimal added salt.

7. Hot Sauce (Low Sodium)

- **Potassium Content:** Many hot sauces are low in potassium, with around 10-20 mg per teaspoon. However, they can be high in sodium, so choose low-sodium options.
- **Uses:** Hot sauce can be added to dishes for extra heat and flavor. Use it sparingly to avoid excessive sodium intake.

8. Greek Yogurt (Plain)

- **Potassium Content:** Plain Greek yogurt contains approximately 200-250 mg of potassium per cup. It's a good source of protein and can be used as a base for sauces and dressings.
- **Uses:** Greek yogurt can be used to make creamy dressings, dips, or as a substitute for sour cream. Opt for plain varieties without added sugars or potassium-based ingredients.

9. Apple Cider Vinegar

- **Potassium Content:** Apple cider vinegar contains minimal potassium, about 10 mg per tablespoon. It adds a tangy flavor to dressings and marinades.
- **Uses:** Apple cider vinegar can be used in salad dressings, marinades, and as a flavor enhancer for vegetables and grains.

10. Fresh Herbs and Spices

- **Potassium Content:** Fresh herbs like basil, chives, and parsley are low in potassium. They can be used to add flavor without increasing potassium levels.
- **Uses:** Fresh herbs can be used in dressings, marinades, and as garnishes to enhance flavor without added sodium or potassium.

11. Hummus (Low-Sodium)

- **Potassium Content:** Hummus typically contains around 200-250 mg of potassium per quarter-cup serving. Look for low-sodium varieties to manage sodium intake.
- **Uses:** Hummus can be used as a dip for vegetables or as a spread on sandwiches. Choose versions with minimal added salt.

12. Mayonnaise (Low Sodium)

- **Potassium Content:** Regular mayonnaise is low in potassium, about 5-10 mg per tablespoon. Choose low-sodium varieties to limit sodium intake.
- **Uses:** Mayonnaise can be used in sandwiches, salads, and dressings. Opt for versions with reduced sodium.

13. Cranberry Sauce (Low-Sugar)

- **Potassium Content:** Low-sugar cranberry sauce contains around 150-200 mg of potassium per quarter-cup serving. Choose versions with reduced sugar to manage overall health.
- **Uses:** Cranberry sauce can be used as a condiment with meats or as a flavoring in various dishes.

When incorporating condiments and sauces into your diet, always check labels for potassium, sodium, and other ingredients. Using these safe options in moderation can help enhance the flavor of your meals while adhering to dietary restrictions and supporting kidney health.

9. Sample Low Potassium Meal Plans

9.1 Breakfast Ideas

Starting your day with a kidney-friendly breakfast can help you manage potassium intake while ensuring you get a nutritious start. Here are some breakfast ideas that are low in potassium and suitable for individuals with kidney disease.

1. Oatmeal with Fresh Berries

- **Ingredients:** Rolled oats, fresh blueberries or strawberries, a splash of almond milk (unsweetened).

- **Potassium Content:** Oatmeal is generally low in potassium, and berries like blueberries and strawberries are lower in potassium compared to other fruits. Almond milk is a good low-potassium alternative to dairy.
- **Preparation:** Cook the rolled oats according to package instructions, then top with fresh berries and a splash of almond milk. You can add a sprinkle of cinnamon for extra flavor.

2. Greek Yogurt with Honey and Chia Seeds

- **Ingredients:** Plain Greek yogurt, a drizzle of honey, chia seeds.
- **Potassium Content:** Greek yogurt, especially when low in potassium, provides protein without excessive potassium. Chia seeds add texture and fiber, while honey provides natural sweetness.
- **Preparation:** Combine Greek yogurt with a drizzle of honey and a teaspoon of chia seeds. Mix well and enjoy.

3. Scrambled Eggs with Spinach

- **Ingredients:** Eggs, fresh spinach, a small amount of olive oil.
- **Potassium Content:** Eggs are low in potassium, and fresh spinach can be used in small quantities. Spinach is higher in potassium, so use it sparingly.
- **Preparation:** Scramble eggs in a pan with a small amount of olive oil. Add a handful of fresh spinach just before the eggs are fully cooked, allowing it to wilt slightly.

4. Whole Wheat Toast with Avocado

- **Ingredients:** Whole wheat bread, half a ripe avocado, a pinch of salt.
- **Potassium Content:** Whole wheat toast is lower in potassium than some other breads. Avocado should be used in moderation as it is higher in potassium, but a small amount is generally acceptable.

- **Preparation:** Toast a slice of whole wheat bread and spread a thin layer of mashed avocado on top. Season with a pinch of salt if desired.

5. Smoothie with Low-Potassium Fruits

- **Ingredients:** Fresh berries (e.g., strawberries, blueberries), almond milk (unsweetened), a small handful of spinach.
- **Potassium Content:** Berries are lower in potassium, and almond milk is a good choice. Spinach should be used sparingly due to its higher potassium content.
- **Preparation:** Blend a small handful of berries with almond milk and a few spinach leaves. Blend until smooth and enjoy.

6. Cottage Cheese with Sliced Pears

- **Ingredients:** Low-fat cottage cheese, fresh pear slices.
- **Potassium Content:** Cottage cheese is low in potassium, and pears are a low-potassium fruit.
- **Preparation:** Serve a portion of low-fat cottage cheese with fresh pear slices on the side.

7. Rice Cakes with Almond Butter

- **Ingredients:** Plain rice cakes, almond butter (unsweetened).
- **Potassium Content:** Rice cakes are low in potassium, and almond butter is a suitable option when used in moderation.
- **Preparation:** Spread a thin layer of unsweetened almond butter on plain rice cakes.

8. Overnight Oats with Almond Milk

- **Ingredients:** Rolled oats, unsweetened almond milk, a touch of maple syrup, a few fresh berries.

- **Potassium Content:** Rolled oats and almond milk are low in potassium. Adding a small amount of fresh berries keeps potassium levels manageable.
- **Preparation:** Combine rolled oats with almond milk and a touch of maple syrup. Refrigerate overnight and top with a few fresh berries before serving.

9. Egg White Omelet with Bell Peppers

- **Ingredients:** Egg whites, diced bell peppers, a small amount of olive oil.
- **Potassium Content:** Egg whites are low in potassium, and bell peppers are a lower-potassium vegetable.
- **Preparation:** Prepare an omelet using egg whites and a small amount of diced bell peppers. Cook with a touch of olive oil for flavor.

10. Plain English Muffin with Low-Fat Cream Cheese

- **Ingredients:** Plain English muffin, low-fat cream cheese.
- **Potassium Content:** English muffins and low-fat cream cheese are both low in potassium.
- **Preparation:** Toast the English muffin and spread a thin layer of low-fat cream cheese on top.

These breakfast ideas provide a range of options that are low in potassium and nutritious, ensuring you start your day on the right foot while adhering to dietary restrictions. Always consider portion sizes and ingredients to align with your specific dietary needs.

9.2 Lunch and Dinner Suggestions

Creating kidney-friendly meals for lunch and dinner involves focusing on low-potassium ingredients while ensuring balanced nutrition. Here are some meal ideas that are both delicious and suitable for individuals managing kidney disease.

1. Grilled Chicken Salad

- **Ingredients:** Grilled chicken breast, mixed greens (e.g., lettuce, spinach in small amounts), cucumbers, bell peppers, olive oil, and balsamic vinegar.
- **Potassium Content:** Chicken breast is low in potassium, and using a variety of low-potassium vegetables like cucumbers and bell peppers adds crunch and nutrition without excessive potassium.
- **Preparation:** Grill chicken breast and slice it. Toss with mixed greens and chopped vegetables. Dress with a light mixture of olive oil and balsamic vinegar.

2. Baked Salmon with Steamed Broccoli

- **Ingredients:** Salmon fillet, lemon juice, fresh herbs (e.g., dill), broccoli.
- **Potassium Content:** Salmon is a good source of protein and omega-3 fatty acids without excessive potassium. Broccoli should be used in moderation due to its higher potassium content.
- **Preparation:** Season salmon with lemon juice and fresh herbs. Bake until cooked through. Serve with steamed broccoli.

3. Turkey and Vegetable Stir-Fry

- **Ingredients:** Ground turkey, bell peppers, snap peas, carrots, garlic, ginger, low-sodium soy sauce.
- **Potassium Content:** Ground turkey is low in potassium, and bell peppers, snap peas, and carrots are lower-potassium vegetables when used in moderation.
- **Preparation:** Cook ground turkey in a pan, then add chopped vegetables and stir-fry with garlic, ginger, and a splash of low-sodium soy sauce.

4. Quinoa and Vegetable Bowl

- **Ingredients:** Quinoa, cherry tomatoes, cucumbers, zucchini, fresh herbs (e.g., parsley), lemon vinaigrette.
- **Potassium Content:** Quinoa is a lower-potassium grain, and the selected vegetables are used in controlled portions.
- **Preparation:** Cook quinoa according to package instructions. Combine with chopped vegetables and fresh herbs. Toss with a lemon vinaigrette.

5. Chicken and Rice Soup

- **Ingredients:** Chicken breast, low-sodium chicken broth, rice, carrots, celery, thyme.
- **Potassium Content:** Chicken breast and rice are low in potassium, and carrots and celery are used in moderate amounts.
- **Preparation:** Simmer chicken breast in low-sodium chicken broth. Add rice, carrots, celery, and thyme. Cook until vegetables and rice are tender.

6. Stuffed Bell Peppers

- **Ingredients:** Bell peppers, ground beef or turkey, rice, diced tomatoes, spices (e.g., cumin, paprika).
- **Potassium Content:** Bell peppers and ground beef or turkey are suitable for a low-potassium diet when used in moderation.
- **Preparation:** Mix cooked ground beef or turkey with rice and diced tomatoes. Stuff the mixture into halved bell peppers. Bake until peppers are tender.

7. Baked Cod with Asparagus

- **Ingredients:** Cod fillet, olive oil, lemon slices, fresh herbs (e.g., rosemary), asparagus.
- **Potassium Content:** Cod is low in potassium, and asparagus is used in moderation.
- **Preparation:** Season cod with olive oil, lemon slices, and fresh herbs. Bake until cooked through. Serve with lightly steamed asparagus.

8. Lentil Soup

- **Ingredients:** Low-sodium vegetable broth, lentils, carrots, celery, bay leaf.
- **Potassium Content:** Lentils are moderate in potassium, so use them in controlled portions. Carrots and celery add flavor without excessive potassium.
- **Preparation:** Simmer lentils in low-sodium vegetable broth with chopped carrots, celery, and a bay leaf until tender.

9. Turkey Lettuce Wraps

- **Ingredients:** Ground turkey, lettuce leaves, diced bell peppers, shredded carrots, a small amount of low-sodium soy sauce.
- **Potassium Content:** Ground turkey is low in potassium, and lettuce, bell peppers, and carrots are used in moderate amounts.
- **Preparation:** Cook ground turkey with diced bell peppers and shredded carrots. Serve in lettuce leaves with a small drizzle of low-sodium soy sauce.

10. Spinach and Feta Stuffed Chicken Breast

- **Ingredients:** Chicken breast, fresh spinach (used in small quantities), feta cheese, garlic.
- **Potassium Content:** Chicken breast is low in potassium, and using a small amount of fresh spinach and feta cheese adds flavor without excessive potassium.
- **Preparation:** Stuff chicken breasts with a mixture of chopped spinach and feta cheese. Bake until chicken is cooked through.

These lunch and dinner suggestions offer a variety of flavors and nutrients while adhering to a low-potassium diet. Always be mindful of portion sizes and ingredient choices to ensure they align with your dietary needs and restrictions.

9.3 Snack Options

Finding satisfying and kidney-friendly snacks is key to managing potassium intake while keeping hunger at bay. Here are some snack ideas that are low in potassium and provide balanced nutrition for individuals with kidney disease.

1. Apple Slices with Almond Butter

- **Ingredients:** Fresh apple slices, almond butter (unsweetened).
- **Potassium Content:** Apples are low in potassium, and almond butter can be used in moderation.
- **Preparation:** Slice an apple and serve with a thin layer of unsweetened almond butter for a crunchy and satisfying snack.

2. Rice Cakes with Cream Cheese

- **Ingredients:** Plain rice cakes, low-fat cream cheese.
- **Potassium Content:** Rice cakes and low-fat cream cheese are both low in potassium.
- **Preparation:** Spread a thin layer of low-fat cream cheese on plain rice cakes.

3. Carrot Sticks with Hummus

- **Ingredients:** Fresh carrot sticks, low-sodium hummus.
- **Potassium Content:** Carrots are lower in potassium, and hummus can be used in controlled portions.
- **Preparation:** Dip fresh carrot sticks into a small serving of low-sodium hummus.

4. Greek Yogurt with Fresh Berries

- **Ingredients:** Plain Greek yogurt, a few fresh strawberries or blueberries.

- **Potassium Content:** Greek yogurt is low in potassium, and berries are lower-potassium fruits.
- **Preparation:** Top a serving of plain Greek yogurt with a few fresh berries for a refreshing snack.

5. Plain Popcorn

- **Ingredients:** Plain popcorn (air-popped), a small amount of olive oil (optional).
- **Potassium Content:** Plain popcorn is low in potassium. Use olive oil sparingly if desired.
- **Preparation:** Air-pop popcorn and enjoy as a low-potassium, high-fiber snack. Avoid adding salt or butter.

6. Celery Sticks with Light Cream Cheese

- **Ingredients:** Fresh celery sticks, light cream cheese.
- **Potassium Content:** Celery is lower in potassium, and light cream cheese can be used in moderation.
- **Preparation:** Spread light cream cheese on fresh celery sticks for a crunchy and creamy snack.

7. Cucumber Slices with Dill Dip

- **Ingredients:** Fresh cucumber slices, dill dip made with Greek yogurt.
- **Potassium Content:** Cucumbers are low in potassium, and Greek yogurt used in the dip is also low in potassium.
- **Preparation:** Slice cucumbers and dip them into a dill-flavored Greek yogurt dip.

8. Hard-Boiled Eggs

- **Ingredients:** Eggs.
- **Potassium Content:** Eggs are low in potassium and provide a good source of protein.
- **Preparation:** Boil eggs, peel, and enjoy as a simple, protein-rich snack.

9. Unsweetened Applesauce

- **Ingredients:** Unsweetened applesauce.
- **Potassium Content:** Applesauce is lower in potassium compared to whole apples.
- **Preparation:** Serve a small portion of unsweetened applesauce as a sweet and satisfying snack.

10. Plain Cottage Cheese with Pineapple

- **Ingredients:** Plain cottage cheese, fresh pineapple chunks.
- **Potassium Content:** Cottage cheese is low in potassium, and pineapple can be used in small amounts.
- **Preparation:** Combine a serving of plain cottage cheese with a few fresh pineapple chunks.

11. Low-Potassium Muffins

- **Ingredients:** Low-potassium ingredients (e.g., white flour, a small amount of blueberries), egg substitute.
- **Potassium Content:** Ensure muffins are made with low-potassium ingredients and in controlled portions.
- **Preparation:** Bake muffins using low-potassium ingredients and enjoy as a treat. Check recipes to ensure they align with dietary restrictions.

12. Smoothie with Low-Potassium Fruits

- **Ingredients:** Fresh berries (e.g., strawberries, blueberries), almond milk (unsweetened).
- **Potassium Content:** Berries and almond milk are both lower in potassium.
- **Preparation:** Blend fresh berries with almond milk for a refreshing and nutritious smoothie.

These snack options offer a variety of flavors and textures while keeping potassium levels in check. Be mindful of portion sizes and ingredient choices to ensure that snacks fit within your dietary guidelines and support kidney health.

10. Practical Tips for Managing a Low Potassium Diet

10.1 Grocery Shopping for Low Potassium Foods

When managing kidney disease, it's important to carefully select foods that are low in potassium. Here's a guide to help you shop for low-potassium foods effectively:

1. Fresh Fruits

- **Examples:** Apples, berries (strawberries, blueberries), grapes, pears.
- **Notes:** These fruits are typically lower in potassium compared to bananas, oranges, and avocados.

2. Vegetables

- **Examples:** Bell peppers, cucumbers, lettuce, radishes, summer squash.
- **Notes:** Use vegetables like carrots and broccoli in moderation due to their higher potassium content.

3. Proteins

- **Examples:** Chicken breast, turkey breast, fish (cod, tilapia), egg whites.
- **Notes:** Opt for fresh, unprocessed proteins. Avoid high-potassium meats and processed options.

4. Grains and Cereals

- **Examples:** White rice, quinoa, white bread, plain rice cakes.

- **Notes:** Choose grains that are lower in potassium and avoid whole grains if they are too high in potassium for your needs.

5. Dairy and Alternatives

- **Examples:** Greek yogurt (plain), almond milk (unsweetened), low-fat cottage cheese.
- **Notes:** Opt for dairy alternatives that are low in potassium and avoid regular milk or cheese if potassium levels are high.

6. Condiments and Sauces

- **Examples:** Olive oil, balsamic vinegar, lemon juice, mustard.
- **Notes:** Use low-potassium condiments and sauces to flavor meals without adding excessive potassium.

7. Snacks

- **Examples:** Plain popcorn, rice cakes, low-potassium muffins.
- **Notes:** Choose snacks that are low in potassium and avoid those with nuts and high-potassium ingredients.

8. Baking and Cooking Essentials

- **Examples:** All-purpose flour, sugar, baking powder.
- **Notes:** Select baking ingredients that are low in potassium and avoid those with high-potassium additives.

9. Beverages

- **Examples:** Water, herbal teas (check for added potassium), almond milk.
- **Notes:** Stick to beverages that are low in potassium and avoid fruit juices or soft drinks with high potassium content.

10. Low-Potassium Convenience Foods

- **Examples:** Low-sodium soups, low-potassium frozen meals.
- **Notes:** Look for convenience foods specifically labeled as low in potassium or low in sodium to manage overall intake.

When shopping, always check labels for potassium content and other nutritional information to ensure they meet your dietary needs. Keeping a list of safe, low-potassium foods can help you make informed choices and maintain a balanced diet.

10.2 Maintaining Nutritional Balance

Maintaining a nutritional balance is crucial for individuals with kidney disease, as it helps ensure you get the necessary nutrients while managing potassium intake. Here are key strategies for achieving and maintaining nutritional balance:

1. Monitor Potassium Intake

- **Key Points:** Focus on consuming low-potassium foods and limit moderate potassium foods. Use a food diary or app to track daily potassium intake and make adjustments as needed.

2. Prioritize Protein Sources

- **Key Points:** Choose high-quality, low-potassium protein sources such as lean poultry, fish, and egg whites. Protein is essential for maintaining muscle mass and overall health.

3. Incorporate Variety

- **Key Points:** Include a variety of fruits, vegetables, grains, and proteins in your diet to ensure you receive a wide range of nutrients. This variety helps prevent deficiencies and promotes overall well-being.

4. Balance Carbohydrates

- **Key Points:** Opt for low-potassium grains like white rice, quinoa, and white bread. Balance carbohydrate intake with protein and healthy fats to maintain energy levels and support metabolic health.

5. Use Herbs and Spices

- **Key Points:** Enhance flavor without adding potassium by using fresh herbs and low-potassium spices. This can make meals more enjoyable and reduce the need for high-sodium seasonings.

6. Stay Hydrated

- **Key Points:** Drink adequate fluids, primarily water, to stay hydrated. If fluid intake needs to be restricted due to kidney function, monitor and adjust according to medical advice.

7. Manage Sodium Intake

- **Key Points:** Reduce sodium intake by avoiding processed foods and using low-sodium alternatives. High sodium levels can exacerbate kidney issues and contribute to high blood pressure.

8. Plan Balanced Meals

- **Key Points:** Plan meals to include a mix of proteins, low-potassium vegetables, and low-potassium grains. Proper meal planning helps maintain balance and prevents nutrient imbalances.

9. Consult a Dietitian

- **Key Points:** Work with a registered dietitian or nutritionist who specializes in kidney disease to create a personalized eating plan. They can provide guidance on meeting nutritional needs while managing potassium and other dietary restrictions.

10. Monitor Health Regularly

- **Key Points:** Regularly check your health status with your healthcare provider. Blood tests can help monitor potassium levels, kidney function, and overall nutritional status to make necessary dietary adjustments.

Maintaining nutritional balance while managing potassium intake requires careful planning and monitoring. By following these strategies, you can support overall health and well-being while adhering to dietary restrictions

10.3 Eating Out on a Low Potassium Diet

Eating out while adhering to a low-potassium diet can be challenging, but with careful planning and mindful choices, you can enjoy meals at restaurants without compromising your dietary restrictions. Here are some tips for dining out on a low-potassium diet:

1. Choose Restaurants Wisely

- **Key Points:** Opt for restaurants that offer customizable menu options or those known for fresh, unprocessed foods. Places with a focus on healthy or vegetarian cuisine often provide more control over ingredients.

2. Review Menus in Advance

- **Key Points:** Check the restaurant's menu online before dining. Look for low-potassium options or dishes that can be easily modified. Contact the restaurant if you have specific dietary questions.

3. Communicate Dietary Needs

- **Key Points:** Inform your server about your dietary restrictions and request modifications to meals to lower potassium content. Ask for dishes to be prepared without high-potassium ingredients.

4. Select Low-Potassium Options

- **Key Points:** Opt for dishes with low-potassium vegetables like bell peppers, cucumbers, or lettuce. Choose proteins like grilled chicken or fish and avoid items with sauces or dressings high in potassium.

5. Be Mindful of Portion Sizes

- **Key Points:** Restaurant portions can be large. Consider sharing a dish, or take half of your meal home to manage portion sizes and control potassium intake.

6. Avoid High-Potassium Ingredients

- **Key Points:** Steer clear of dishes with potatoes, tomatoes, or high-potassium sauces. Instead, choose dishes that feature ingredients like rice, pasta, or grains that are lower in potassium.

7. Request Cooking Modifications

- **Key Points:** Ask for dishes to be prepared with minimal salt and low-potassium seasonings. Request that vegetables be steamed or grilled instead of sautéed or roasted.

8. Make Smart Beverage Choices

- **Key Points:** Opt for water, herbal teas, or beverages that are low in potassium. Avoid fruit juices, which can be high in potassium, and limit or skip alcoholic drinks.

9. Monitor Ingredients

- **Key Points:** Be aware of hidden sources of potassium in dishes, such as those in sauces, dressings, or seasoning blends. Ask for ingredient lists or preparation methods if necessary.

10. Plan Ahead for Special Occasions

- **Key Points:** For special events or celebrations, plan ahead by contacting the restaurant to discuss your dietary needs or by reviewing the menu thoroughly to make the best choices.

By following these tips, you can navigate dining out while managing a low-potassium diet. Preparation and communication are key to ensuring you enjoy your meals without compromising your health goals.

11. Conclusion

11.1 Encouragement for Adopting a Low Potassium Diet

Adopting a low-potassium diet can be a significant lifestyle change, but it is a crucial step in managing kidney disease and maintaining overall health. Here are some encouraging thoughts and tips to help you embrace this dietary adjustment with a positive mindset:

1. Focus on the Benefits

- **Key Points:** A low-potassium diet helps manage kidney function, reduce symptoms, and prevent complications. By adhering to this diet, you are taking proactive steps to support your health and well-being.

2. Celebrate Small Wins

- **Key Points:** Recognize and celebrate your successes, whether it's trying a new low-potassium recipe or successfully navigating a dining-out experience. Every positive step you take is a victory.

3. Explore New Foods and Recipes

- **Key Points:** A low-potassium diet opens the door to discovering new foods and recipes. Embrace this opportunity to explore a variety of fruits, vegetables, and dishes that you might not have tried before.

4. Seek Support and Guidance

- **Key Points:** Reach out to healthcare professionals, dietitians, and support groups for guidance and encouragement. They can provide valuable information, share tips, and help you stay motivated.

5. Plan and Prepare

- **Key Points:** Planning meals and snacks ahead of time can make adhering to a low-potassium diet easier and less stressful. Meal prepping and creating a shopping list can help you stay organized and focused.

6. Embrace Flexibility

- **Key Points:** Understand that flexibility is key. It's okay to make adjustments and find balance as you learn what works best for you. Adaptation is part of the process, and it's important to be kind to yourself.

7. Stay Positive and Patient

- **Key Points:** Adopting a new diet takes time and effort. Stay positive and patient with yourself as you navigate this change. Progress may be gradual, but every effort counts towards your health goals.

8. Involve Family and Friends

- **Key Points:** Share your dietary goals with family and friends. Their support can make a big difference in your journey, and they can help you make low-potassium choices during meals and social gatherings.

9. Keep Learning

- **Key Points:** Continuously educate yourself about low-potassium foods and nutrition. Staying informed will empower you to make better choices and feel more confident in managing your diet.

10. Focus on the Positive Impact

- **Key Points:** Remind yourself of the positive impact a low-potassium diet has on your health. Improved kidney function, reduced symptoms, and overall well-being are all significant benefits of sticking to your dietary plan.

Adopting a low-potassium diet is a commitment to your health and quality of life. Embrace the change with a positive attitude, and remember that every small step you take contributes to your overall health and well-being.